TH ESS

HANDBOOK

JAMES PERCIVAL

 Credence Publications

The Essiac Handbook

Copyright © 1994
James Percival

The right of James Percival to be identified as the Author of the
Work has been asserted by him in accordance with the
Copyright, Designs and Patents Act 1988

First published in 1994
by Bernard Barbieux Associates

Published in the United Kingdom with permission by

Credence Publications
PO Box 3
TONBRIDGE
Kent TN12 9ZY
UK

1st Ed. VS

TABLE OF CONTENTS

FOREWORD

For years now I have been interested in alternative treatments for debilitating diseases which seem to threaten all of us, such as cancer, AIDS, multiple sclerosis, lupus, chronic fatigue, Alzheimer's, etc. In the course of pursuing this interest, I was enthusiastic about some treatment methods, which appeared successful. However, this enthusiasm was nothing compared to the enthusiasm and excitement I felt when I discovered the story of Rene Caisse's herbal remedy, which she called Essiac.

The story of the development of Essiac, the struggle to get this knowledge out to the public, and the information available about the documented cases of thousands of persons recovering from cancer and other diseases is, I believe, a story you will want to know.

Knowledge of Essiac may change your life. It will give you the knowledge to make more informed decisions for yourself and your loved ones concerning cancer, AIDS, and other prevalent diseases which threaten every family. I am hoping this booklet will also give many of you enough knowledge and interest in the four common herbs of Rene's formula so that you will seek out herbalists who can teach you how to identify, collect and process your own Essiac.

This handbook is written with the goal of getting the word out to as many people as possible about Rene's discovery. If you are as enthusiastic about Essiac as I am, I am sure that you will find yourself mentioning it to many of your friends and acquaintances. You may also find yourself taking Rene's herbal remedy daily as a preventative and detoxifier.

In summary, the information contained herein is offered to you in the spirit of love and brotherhood. We hope you accept it as such, process the information, and pass it along in the spirit of love and brotherhood! In today's society, we live with a lot of fear. It is my hope that your knowledge of Rene's work may better assist you to live without fear concerning several of our most dangerous diseases.

I am not a physician, I am a researcher. I make no claims that Essiac will cure you. I am simply reporting the information which is available in other books and magazine articles. Make your own conclusions. Consult your doctor.

James Percival

DEDICATION

This handbook is dedicated to the Native American herbalists and elders whose wisdom and understanding of the earth's natural products led to the development of the Rene Caisse herbal formula known as Essiac.

This handbook is also dedicated to Dr. Gary l. Glum, whose courageous struggle brought the knowledge of Essiac to us.

BACKGROUND

Rene Caisse was a nurse in Canada. In 1923 she observed that one of her doctor's patients, a woman with terminal cancer, made a complete recovery. Enquiring into the matter, Rene found that the woman had cured herself with a herbal remedy which was given to her by an Ojibway Indian herbalist. Rene visited the medicine man, and he freely presented her with his tribe's formula. The formula consisted of four common herbs. They were blended and cooked in a fashion which caused the concoction apparently to have greater medicinal potency than

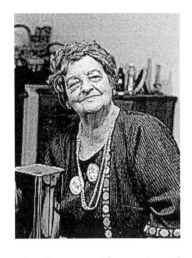

any of the four herbs themselves. The four herbs were Sheep Sorrel, Burdock Root, Slippery Elm Bark, and Rhubarb Root.

With her doctor's permission, Rene began to administer the herbal remedy to other terminal cancer patients, who had been given up by the medical profession as incurable. Most recovered. Rene then began to collect the herbs herself, prepare the remedy in her own kitchen, and treat hundreds of cancer cases. She found that Essiac, as she named the herbal remedy (her own name backwards), could not undo the effects of severe damage to the life support organs. In such cases however, the pain of the illness was alleviated and the life of the patient often extended longer than predicted. In other cases, where the life support organs had not been severely damaged, cure was complete, and the patients sometimes lived another 35 or 40 years. Some are still alive today.

Rene selflessly dedicated herself to helping these patients. She continued to treat hundreds of patients from her home. She did not charge for her services. Donations were her only income. They barely kept her above the poverty line. Over the years, word of her work began to spread. The Canadian medical establishment did not take kindly to this nurse administering this remedy directly to anyone with cancer who requested her help. Thus began many years of harassment and persecution by the Canadian Ministry of Health and Welfare. Word of this struggle was carried throughout Canada by newspapers.

The newspaper coverage of Rene's work began to make her famous throughout Canada. Word was also spread by the families of those healed by Essiac.

Eventually the Royal Cancer Commission became interested in her work. They undertook to study Essiac. In 1937 the Royal Cancer Commission conducted hearings on Essiac. Much testimony was furnished that Essiac was a cure for cancer.

Eventually the Canadian Parliament, prodded by newspaper coverage and the widespread support generated by Rene by former patients and grateful families, voted in 1938 on legislation to legalise the use of Essiac. Fifty-five thousand signatures were collected on a petition presented to the parliament. The vote was close, but Essiac failed by three votes to be approved as an officially sanctioned treatment for cancer.

The complete story of Rene Caisse's life and struggles is told in a book written by Dr. Gary L. Glum, entitled *The Calling of an Angel*. It tells of the documented recoveries of thousands of cancer patients who had been certified in writing by their doctors as incurable. Rene continued her work for 40 years until her death in 1978. Rene had entrusted her formula to several friends, one of whom passed the formula along to Dr. Glum.

Of interest is that, in the 1960's, Rene Caisse worked with the well-known Brusch Clinic in Massachusetts. Dr. Charles A. Brusch was the personal physician for President John F. Kennedy. After 10 years of research into Essiac, Dr Brusch made the following statement: *"Essiac is a cure for cancer, period. All studies done at laboratories in the United States and Canada support this conclusion."* A testimonial letter from Dr. Brusch is included in this handbook.

Further details are explained in Dr. Glum's book. Instructions on how to order a copy of the book are contained in this handbook. Dr. Glum also distributes, free of charge, the complete formula for Essiac along with instructions on how to brew it. This information is also contained in this handbook. We are indebted to Dr. Glum for his work. He has undergone significant sacrifice to get this information to us. Dr. Glum has also been harassed by his government for his efforts to inform us about Essiac. We trust he is somehow recompensed and rewarded for the losses he has incurred whilst working to spread the word of Rene Caisse's herbal formula.

WHAT ESSIAC IS

Rene Caisse's herbal formula contains four commonly existing herbs:

Sheep Sorrel (*Rumex acetosella*)

The leaves of young Sheep Sorrel plants were popular as a cooking dressing and addition to salads in France several hundred years ago. Indians also use Sheep Sorrel leaves as a tasty seasoning for meat dishes. They also baked it into their bread. Thus it is both an herb and a food.

Sheep Sorrel belongs to the buckwheat family. Common names for Sheep Sorrel are field sorrel, red top sorrel, sour grass and dog eared sorrel. It should not be confused with Garden Sorrel (*Rumex acetosa*).

Sheep Sorrel grows wild throughout most of the world. It seeks open pastures, rocky areas, and the shoulders of country roads. It is considered to be a common weed throughout the U.S. It thrives with little moisture, and is a good indicator of acidic soils.

The entire Sheep Sorrel plant may be harvested to be used in Essiac. Alternatively, just the leaves and stems may be harvested, and this allows the plants to be 're-harvested' later. The plant portion of the Sheep Sorrel may be harvested throughout the spring, summer and fall, to be taken early in the morning after the dew has evaporated, or late in the afternoon. Always harvest on a sunny day, as the plants need several days after a rain in which to dry properly. Harvest the leaves and stem before the flowers begin to form, since at this stage, all of the energy of the plant is in the leaves.

Roots may be harvested in the fall, when the energy of the plant is concentrated in the roots. Never collect more than a year's supply of Sheep Sorrel, as it loses its potency when stored longer.

Burdock Root (*Arctium lappa*)

The roots, young stems, and seeds of the Burdock plant are edible. Young stalks are boiled to be eaten like asparagus. Raw stems and young leaves are eaten in salads. Parts of the Burdock plant are eaten in China, Hawaii, and among the Native American cultures on this continent. It is both an herb and a food.

The Burdock is a member of the thistle family. Remember the last time you cleaned cockle burrs from your clothing when returning from the woods or meadow? You had just run up against this very friendly and helpful plant. It is a common pasture weed throughout North America. It prefers damp soils.

The first years the Burdock plant produces only green leafy growth. It is during the second year that it produces the long sturdy stems with those little burrs.

The root of the Burdock plant is harvested from only the first-year plants. The roots are about an inch wide, and up to three feet long. As with the Sheep Sorrel, the roots should only be harvested in the fall when the plant energy is concentrated in the roots.

Slippery Elm (*Ulmus fulva*)
The inner bark of the Slippery Elm tree has a long history of use as a food supplement and herbal remedy. Pioneers also knew of it as a survival food. The powdered bark has long been used, and is still being used today, as a food additive and food extender, rich in vitamin and mineral content. Thus it also is a food.

The Slippery Elm gives much shade and is a favoured ornamental tree. It is found throughout Canada and the United States. Only the inner bark of the Slippery Elm is used to make Essiac. Reliable supplies of Slippery Elm can be purchased in powdered form, and this is probably easier and preferable to harvesting it yourself. Should you wish to harvest your own Slippery Elm, strip the bark from branches, rather than from the main trunk system of the tree so that you do not damage the tree.

Turkey Rhubarb (*Rheum palmatum*)
We have all eaten Rhubarb. Its red, bittersweet stems are to be found in supermarket produce shelves each spring. We also eat rhubarb pie, jams and pudding. The Turkey Rhubarb is a member of the rhubarb family with roots which contain a particularly strong and desirable potency.

The Turkey Rhubarb grows in China. The roots are harvested when the plants are at least six years old. This imported product has more potency than our native rhubarb. Rene Caisse began her Essiac work using the domestic rhubarb root, later discovering that the imported variety was more potent. However, most of the Turkey Rhubarb, which is now imported into this country, is irradiated, which destroys many of its properties. So native rhubarb is now once again the rhubarb of choice for your Essiac blend.

Notes: Look for evening classes on herbs and herb identification. Seek out herbalists, preferably qualified in pharmacognosy, who are willing to educate you on plant identity, harvesting techniques, plant drying and processing. Do not collect herbs from areas where insecticides or herbicides have been used. You want only organic herbs!

THE FORMULA

The original formula, as given by Rene Caisse, is listed below. We are reprinting Rene's exact instructions for a two-gallon supply, although you would probably not need such a large amount at one time. A smaller amount is offered in the mail order dried herbal package, which makes 1/2 gallon of Essiac (which is a two-week or four-week supply, depending upon whether you take it once or twice daily).

Ingredients (parts by weight):
52 parts: Burdock Root (cut or dried)
16 parts: Sheep Sorrel (powdered)
1 part: Turkey Rhubarb (powdered) or 2 parts domestic Rhubarb
4 parts: Slippery Elm (powdered)

This is the basic four-herb formula which was presented to the Canadian medical authorities for evaluation in 1937. Later in her life, while working with Dr. Charles Brusch in Cambridge, Massachusetts, Rene added small amounts of four other herbs to her basic four-herb formula. As provided to us by a woman who worked with Rene, and who was given the formula by Rene, these extra four herbs were added as follows: Kelp (2 parts), Red Clover (1 part), Blessed Thistle (1 part),

Watercress (0.4 parts). We consider the addition of these four extra herbs optional.

Supplies Needed:
One 4-gallon stainless steel pot with lid.
One 3-gallon stainless steel pot with lid.
One stainless steel fine mesh double strainer, funnel & spatula.
12 or more 16 oz. sterilized amber glass bottles with airtight caps, or suitable substitutes.

Preparation:

1. Mix dry ingredients thoroughly. Place herbs in a plastic bag and shake vigorously. Herbs are light sensitive; keep stored in a cool dark place.
2. Bring 2 gallons of sodium-free distilled water to a rolling boil in the 4-gallon pot (with lid on). Should take approximately 30 minutes at sea level.
3. Stir in 1 cup of dry ingredients. Replace lid and continue to boil for 10 minutes.
4. Turn off stove. Scrape down the sides of the pot with the spatula and stir mixture thoroughly. Replace the lid.
5. Allow the pot to remain closed for 12 hours. Then turn the stove to the highest setting and heat almost to a boil (approximately 20 minutes). Do not let boil.
6. Turn off the stove. Strain the liquid into the 3-gallon pot. Clean the 4-gallon pot and strainer. Then strain the filtered liquid back into the 4-gallon pot.
7. Use the funnel to pour the hot liquid into sterilised bottles immediately, and tighten the caps. After the bottles have cooled, retighten the caps.
8. Refrigerate. Rene's herbal drink contains no preservative agents. If mold should develop, discard the bottle immediately.

Caution: All bottles and caps must be sterilised after use if you plan to reuse them for Essiac. Bottle caps must be washed and rinsed thoroughly, and may be cleaned with a 3% solution of food-grade hydrogen peroxide (purchased in health food stores). To make a 3% solution, mix 1 ounce of 35% food grade hydrogen peroxide with 11 ounces of sodium-free distilled water. Allow to soak for 5 minutes, rinse and dry. If food-grade hydrogen peroxide is not available, use one half teaspoon of Clorox to one gallon of distilled water.

INSTRUCTIONS FOR USE

1. Keep refrigerated.
2. Shake bottle well before using.
3. May be taken either cold from the bottle, or warmed (never microwave).
4. Once or twice daily, take 4 tablespoons (2 ounces) on an empty stomach at least 2 hours after eating.
5. Cancer and AIDS sufferers, or other ill people, may wish twice daily to take 4 tablespoons (2 ounces), once in the morning, 5 minutes before eating and once in the evening, at least 2 hours after eating.

Note: Stomach cancer patients must dilute the herbal drink with an equal amount of sodium-free distilled water. Many people have reported that Rene's drink works well to detoxify the body and have taken it as a detoxification program.

Precaution: Some doctors advise against taking the herbal formula while pregnant.

Recommendation: Rene reported that the twelve-hour brewing process is essential for Essiac to develop its proper potency. Essiac is being offered to the public in teabags and homeopathic drops. We do not recommend them. They may work, but they are not what Rene Caisse used, nor have we seen evidence that they work.

WHAT IT DOES

The components of Rene's herbal drink interact to have an amazing effect upon the human body. The chemicals, minerals and vitamins appear to act synergistically to produce a variety of healing agents.

Sheep Sorrel:

Sorrel plants have been a folk remedy for cancer for centuries both in Europe and America. Sheep Sorrel has been observed by researchers to break down tumours and to alleviate some chronic conditions and degenerative diseases.

It contains high amounts of vitamins A and B complex, C,D,E,K,P, and vitamin U. It is also rich in minerals, including calcium, chlorine, iron, magnesium, silicon, sodium, sulphur and has trace amount of copper, iodine, manganese and zinc. The combination of these vitamins and minerals nourishes the glands of the body. Sheep Sorrel also contains carotenoids and chlorophyll, citric, malic, oxalic, tannic and tartaric acids.

The chlorophyll carries oxygen throughout the bloodstream. Cancer cells do not live in the presence of oxygen. Sheep Sorrel may also help to:

- reduce the damage of radiation burns
- increase resistance to x-rays
- improve the vascular system, heart function, intestines and lungs
- aid in the removal of foreign deposits from the walls of the blood vessels
- purify the liver and stimulate the growth of new tissue
- reduce inflammation of the pancreas and stimulate the growth of new tissue
- raise the oxygen level of tissue cells

Sheep Sorrel is viewed as the primary healing herb in Essiac.

Burdock Root:

For centuries Burdock has been used throughout the world to cure illness and disease. The root of the Burdock is regarded by many as a powerful blood purifier. It may help to clear congestion in respiratory, lymphatic, urinary and circulatory systems. It may also assist in promoting the flow of bile and eliminating excess fluid in the body. It may help to stimulate the elimination of toxic wastes and relieve liver malfunctions, and improve digestion. It may also play a part in assisting the removal of infection from the urinary tract, the liver, and the gall bladder. It may also assist in expelling toxins through the skin and urine. It has been regarded as beneficial against arthritis, rheumatism and sciatica.

Burdock Root contains vitamins A, B complex, C, E and P. It contains high amounts of chromium, cobalt, iron, magnesium, phosphorus, potassium, silicon and zinc and lesser amounts of calcium, copper, manganese and selenium. Much of the Burdock Root's curative power is attributed to its principal ingredient of Unulin, which may help to strengthen vital organs, especially the liver, pancreas and spleen.

Slippery Elm Inner Bark:

Slippery Elm Bark is widely known throughout the world as a herbal remedy. As a tonic, it is renowned for its ability to soothe and strengthen the organs, tissues, and mucous membranes, especially the lungs and stomach. It may help promote the fast healing of cuts, burns, ulcers and wounds. It mat also help revitalise the entire body.

It contains as its primary ingredient, a mucilage, as well as quantities of gallic acid, phenols, starches, sugars and vitamins A, B, complex, C, K, and P. It contains large amounts of calcium and selenium and trace amounts of iron, phosphorous, silicon and zinc. Slippery Elm Bark is known among herbalists for its ability to cleanse, heal and strengthen the body.

Rhubarb:

Rhubarb, also a well-known herb, has been used worldwide since 220BC as a medicine. The Rhubarb root is reported to exert a gentle laxative action by stimulating the secretion of bile into the intestines. It may also help stimulate the gall duct to expel toxic waste matter, thus purging the body of waste bile and food. As a result of this detoxifying action, the liver may be cleansed and chronic liver problems relieved.

Rhubarb root contains vitamin A and many of the B complex, C, and P. Its high mineral content includes calcium, chlorine, copper, iodine, iron, magnesium, manganese, phosphorous, potassium, silicon, sodium, sulphur and zinc.

REPORTED BENEFITS OF ESSIAC

A number of well-researched and -referenced books have been written on the subject of Essiac (shown in the back of this booklet). In this literature, the authors report the following therapeutic activity for this remedy:

1. Prevents the build up of fatty deposits in artery walls, heart, kidney and liver.
2. Regulates cholesterol levels by transforming sugar and fat into energy.
3. Destroys parasites in the digestive system and throughout the body.
4. Counteracts the effects of aluminium, lead and mercury poisoning.
5. Strengthens and tightens muscles, organs and tissues.
6. Makes bones, joints ligaments, lungs and membranes strong and flexible, less vulnerable to stress or stress injuries.
7. Nourishes and stimulates the brain and nervous system.
8. Promotes the absorption of fluids in the tissues.
9. Removes toxic accumulations in the fat, lymph, bone marrow, bladder, and alimentary canals.
10. Neutralises acids, absorbs toxins in the bowel and eliminates both.
11. Clears the respiratory channels by dissolving and expelling mucus.
12. Relieves the liver of its burden of detoxification by converting fatty toxins into water-soluble substances that can then be easily eliminated through the kidneys.
13. Assists the liver to produce lecithin, which forms part of the myelin sheath, a white, fatty material that encloses nerve fibres.
14. Reduces, perhaps eliminates, heavy metal deposits in tissues (especially those surrounding the joints) to reduce inflammation and stiffness.
15. Improves the function of the pancreas and spleen by increasing the effectiveness of insulin.
16. Purifies the blood.
17. Increases red cell production and keeps them from rupturing.
18. Increases the body's ability to utilise oxygen by raising oxygen level in the tissue cell.

19. Maintains the balance between potassium and sodium within the body so that the fluid inside and outside each cell is regulated: in this way cells are nourished with nutrients and are also cleansed.
20. Converts calcium and potassium oxalates into harmless forms by making them solvent in the urine. Regulates the amount of oxalic acid delivered to the kidneys, thus reducing the risk of stone formation in the gall bladder, kidneys or urinary tract.
21. Protects against toxins entering the brain.
22. Protects the body against radiation and x-rays.
23. Relieves pain, increases the appetite and provides more energy along with a sense of well-being.
24. Speeds up wound healing by regenerating the damaged area.
25. Increases the production of antibodies like lymphocytes and T-cells in the thymus gland, which is the defence of our immune system.
26. Inhibits and possibly destroys benign growths and tumours.

CHRONIC FATIGUE,
LUPUS, ALZHEIMERS, ETC.

We have found Essiac to be very helpful to many people with Chronic Fatigue Syndrome, Lupus, Multiple Sclerosis and Alzheimer's. We have also witnessed very rapid recoveries among chronic fatigue sufferers. Usually they report a dramatic increase in energy. Some Multiple Sclerosis sufferers had less dramatic but steady improvements in their conditions. One lady put her crutches away after taking Essiac for three months. Alzheimer's sufferers have reported improvements. Some with Arthritis have reported improvement, although apparently not all arthritic sufferers are helped by Essiac.

It appears that Essiac's actions to remove heavy metals, detoxify the body, restore energy levels and rebuild the immune system all act to restore the body to a level where it is better able to defeat the illness in question. In other words, Essiac seems to help in the rebuilding of the immune system and improves the illness defeating ability of the body so that it can then rid itself of the illness.

ESSIAC AND AIDS

In 1993, Dr. Gary Glum worked with an AIDS project in Los Angeles. The project had sent 179 AIDS patients home to die. They had pneumocystis carinii and histoplasmosis and were all underweight.

The project gave Dr. Glum five of these patients to work with. He took them off AZT and put them on a protocol, taking 2 ounces of Essiac three times a day. By February of 1994, all of the other patients had died. Dr. Glum's five patients were still alive. They were exercising, eating three meals a day, their weights were back to normal and they had no appearance of illness.

AN ENDORSEMENT BY DR. WHITAKER, M.D.

Dr. Julian Whitaker publishes a very informative and enlightening monthly newsletter named *Health and Healing*. It has 430,000 subscribers. In his November 1995 issue, he had an article entitled "What I Would Do If I Had Cancer". He states that if he had cancer he personally would follow a regime which included Essiac Tea.

Dr. Whitaker has over twenty years' experience. He has written five major health books: *Reversing Heart Disease, Reversing Diabetes, Reversing Health Risks, A Guide to Natural Healing* and *Is Heart Surgery Necessary?* Dr. Whitaker directs the Whitaker Wellness Institute in Newport Beach, California, which has treated thousands of patients. Should you desire information about subscribing to his newsletter, call (800) 705-5559.

I highly recommend this newsletter to anyone who has a serious illness and wishes to become more knowledgeable about the complete range of healing modalities available. He also proscribes a 7-step, 30-day wellness program "that will turn your life around".

QUOTES FROM RENE CAISSE

"Though I worked each day from 9am to 9pm, my work was so absorbing there was no sense of fatigue. My waiting room was a place of happiness where people exchanged their experiences and shared their hope. After a few treatments, patients seemed to throw off their depression, fear and distress. Their outlook became optimistic and as their pain decreased, they became happy and talkative."

19

"I could see the changes in some of the patients. A number of them, presented to me by their doctors after everything known to medical science had been tried and failed, were literally carried into my clinic for their first treatment. To later see these same people walk in on their own, after only five or six treatments, more than repaid me for all my endeavours. I have helped thousands of such people. I offered the treatment at no charge."

"Most importantly, and this was verified in animal tests conducted at the Brusch Medical Centre and other laboratories, it was discovered that one of the most dramatic effects of taking this remedy was its affinity for drawing all of the cancer cells which had spread, back to the original site at which point the tumour would first harden, then later soften until it vanished altogether. In other cases, the tumour would decrease in size to where it could be surgically removed with minimal complications."

DISCLAIMER

We are not permitted, nor do we, in this handbook make any claims that Rene Caisse's formula will cure any disease. We have only gathered together in this easy-to-read handbook much of the already published information that is available to the general public about Rene's herbal remedy so that you may better make informed decisions. The documents which were used to compile this handbook are listed in the bibliography. Please consult your physician before using Rene Caisse's herbal remedy.

TESTIMONIALS

CHARLES A BRUSCH, M.D.
15 GROZIER ROAD
CAMBRIDGE, MA 02138

TO WHOM IT MAY CONCERN:
Many years have gone by since I first experienced the use of ESSIAC with my patients who were suffering from many varied forms of cancer.

I personally monitored the use of this old therapy along with Rene Caisse R.N., whose many successes were widely reported. Rene worked with me at my medical clinic in Cambridge, Massachusetts where, under the supervision of 18 of my medical doctors on staff, she proceeded with a series of treatments on terminal cancer patients and laboratory mice. Together we refined and perfected her formula.

On mice it has been shown to cause a decided recession of the mass and a definite change in cell formation. Clinically, on patients suffering from pathologically proven cancer, it reduces pain and causes a recession in growth. Patients gained weight and showed a great improvement in their general health. Their elimination improved considerably and their appetite became whetted.

Remarkably beneficial results were obtained even on those cases at the "end of the road", where it proved to prolong life and the "quality" of that life. In some cases, if the tumour didn't disappear, it could be surgically removed after ESSIAC with less risk of metastases resulting in new outbreaks.

Haemorrhage has been rapidly brought under control in many difficult cases, open lesions of lip and breast respond to treatment, and patients with cancer of the stomach have returned to normal activity among many other remembered cases. Also, intestinal burns from radiation were healed and damage replaced, and it was found to greatly improve whatever the condition.

All the patient cases were diagnosed by reputable physicians and surgeons. I do know that I have witnessed in my clinic, and know of many other cases, where ESSIAC was the therapy used - a treatment which brings about restoration through destroying the tumour tissue and improving the mental outlook which re-establishes physiological function.

I endorse this therapy even today for I have in fact cured my own cancer, the original site of which was the lower bowel, through ESSIAC alone. My last complete examination, when I was examined throughout the intestinal tract while hospitalized (August, 1989) for a hernia problem, revealed no sign of malignancy. Medical documents validate this. I have taken ESSIAC every day since my diagnosis (1984) and my recent examination has given me a clear bill of health.

I remained a partner with Rene Caisse until her death in 1978 and was the only person who had her complete trust and to whom she confided her knowledge and "know-how" of what she named "ESSIAC."

Others have imitated, but a minor success rate should never be accepted when the true therapy is available.

Executed as a legal document.

Charles A. Brusch, M.D.

Signed, Sealed and Delivered
in the Presence of

Witness:

Address: 2360 Massachusetts Avenue
Cambridge, MA 02140
Occupation: Banker

Date: April 11, 1990

Notary

My Commission expires:

William E. Moriarty
Notary Public
My Commission Expires Oct. 5, 1990

22

In the fall of 1992, my mother, who lives in Ohio, was told that her throat and lung cancer had reached the point that she only had ninety days left to live. My sister and I began to help her straighten out her affairs. I heard about Essiac. I sent her some. She drank it for two months. On December 22, she went back to visit the doctor. He thought that she was coming in to say goodbye. When he checked her she was in total remission. I am a nurse, and I have kept her x-rays as proof of her recovery.

Ellen Broderick
Winter Springs, Florida

I started taking your Essiac several months ago. The results have been profound and dramatic. Thank you.

John Tolleson
Columbus, Ohio

My uncle had lung cancer. They gave him six months to live. He started taking Essiac. That was four years ago. He is convinced the Essiac saved him.

Rhonda M.
Harrison, Ohio

My friend Joe Roberts was in a very bad way with Lupus. He could hardly move about. Some thought he was close to death. I gave him two bottles of herbal tea (Essiac). He improved, and started taking Essiac regularly. Within a month he looked like a new man, and appeared completely healed.

Marsha Mylander
Orlando, Florida

I had prostate cancer. My doctor gave me six months. I took Essiac as well as several other natural cures. My prostate cancer is gone.

A liquor store manager,
Orlando, Florida

My husband has been through every treatment for his illness, and I am now trying Essiac tea. I thought I would try it first for my various aches and pains, stress, etc. I believe it has done

wonders for me so I have started giving him the tea. It won't hurt and maybe his life will be better. A friend of mine has liver cancer and even though the oncologist gave him six months, he is now going on two years and says the only thing he takes is Essiac tea. Believe me, he is living proof of its success for him.

Betty at
MPIP Bulletin Board
July 18, 1997

I met a friend at a seminar. He told me about Essiac. I had a cancerous condition in my female organs which was causing me a lot of pain. I took the Essiac, my pain went away, and I am now free of cancer. God bless you. My eyes are now opened up to the value of natural healing systems, and I spend a lot of time preaching this new religion to my friends.

Marjorie L.
Stuart, Florida

I am 71 years old. I have had a very rare illness for twenty years. The medical people don't know what causes it, and they don't have a cure. It's called Cogan's Syndrome. It has destroyed my hearing in both ears, caused a lot of vertigo, a lot of aches and pains, and has damaged my heart. Most of my life I've had several colds every year and usually a case of flu. In January of 1996, the flu turned into pneumonia. That was when I decided to give your herbal Essiac Tea a try.

I am happy to tell you that since I began using your Essiac I have not had a cold or a sign of flu. I do believe that it has helped my recovery from pneumonia. I plan to continue its use. I drink 2 ounces about three times a week.

Calvin Goranson
299 Lake Mamie Rd.
Deland Fl 32724

My brother-in-law gave me a bottle of Essiac herbal tea to try as a preventative measure. I enjoyed the taste. Soon realized a twenty-year stomach problem was gone, and it gives me an all-round better feeling. I am 60 years old and I work 7 days a week.

My nephew in Wisconsin learned he had cancer. He is unable to take chemo because of other health problems. He takes your tea faithfully. One year later all is in remission. Our family also uses organic sea salt. My wife used to have water retention. No longer has a problem there. We enjoy your products and keep up the good work!

Robert W. Heath
9539 Stevenson Rd.
Fenwick MI 48834

I had prostate cancer. On August 10, 1994 I was given chemotherapy. I never told the doctor that I was taking Essiac and as a result the PSA rating went well below 0 (zero). I took the combination for 15 months and when it held below zero I quit the chemotherapy. Since then the PSA readings went like this:

October:	0.15
April:	0.37
October:	0.58
April:	0.73

I am continuing taking the Essiac.

Paul Roche
East Haven,
Connectecut

I have multiple sclerosis. My friend Kelly started me on Essiac. After three months I was able to put my crutches away. After a year, I walk with only a slight limp.

Barbara Johnson,
Apopka, FL

I am in my fifties. It seems as if all my life I have had the flu at least once each year, and a bad cold for several times each year. It was like you could block out 1 to 2 months of each year when I would be laid up with the flu or a bad cold. I started taking Essiac five years ago. Since that time I have not had the flu, and only had a cold once (I think that the cold was part of a detoxification process). I am sure Essiac did this for me.

M.M.
Orlando, Florida

My brother was diagnosed one year ago with very, very severe leukemia. His doctors gave him chemotherapy for four weeks. The chemo made him look deathly ill. My sister and I were appalled. He looked like death itself. This large man who was over 6 feet tall, lay in his hospital bed in a fetal position, shaking from the chemotherapy.

The doctors told him that he would die in hospital if he stayed, or he could go home and die. My sister is a nurse, and she was determined to save my brother. She knew of the herbal remedy for cancer called Essiac. She asked the doctor to approve bringing Essiac into the hospital to give to our brother. The doctor felt that there was nothing else he could do, so he paved the way with the medical authorities.

My brother began taking Essiac and 10 drops of Pau D' Arco herbal formula each day, once in the morning and once in the evening. His blood count was at 4,800 (10,000 is normal). Within one week of the Essiac treatment he was not only alive, his blood count was at 10,800. In one more week his blood count was up to 14,000 - 4,000 higher than normal.

My brother began his Essiac treatments in August, 1992. He was so healthy by the next January that he and his wife went on a four-month cruise around the world. It is now August 1993, and he is very healthy, active and robust. I have to withhold my name because I do not want a lot of people calling me about his experience. I love my brother very much, we are very close, and I just thank God for simple things like Essiac, and the people all over who prayed for his recovery.

Name withheld by request

I have a friend from West Virginia who has had rheumatoid arthritis for over 9 years. In May I gave her some of my Essiac. She liked it and began taking it regularly. Within 2 weeks she felt great relief from her pain. Within 2 months she could raise her arms full length over her head, something she had not been able to do for 9 years. She just went to Ireland to visit her relatives, and she took some Essiac with her to give to them

Alice Bailey
Winter Springs, Florida

Several years ago, I escorted my mother to the outpatient clinic of a local hospital to have a small lump removed from her parotid gland on the left side of her face. What a shock when the doctors found advanced lymphoma cancer throughout her body. I began researching volumes of books looking for some unknown answer. A program of nutritional supplementation and natural food diet was begun, in addition to chiropractic care, positive thought and humour therapy.

It was extremely tense as the doctors began chemotherapy. In fact mother was taken to the emergency room six times that first month. Being 80, it was probably her strong heart that kept her alive and with me to tell her story today. Dancing and teaching others to stay well through dance has kept her going strong all her life.

Letters with prayers for her improved health poured in and a friend sent an article about Essiac tea. Hopeful that this herbal formula could somehow help, I went searching for the ingredients, brewed the tea, and added it to her growing list of nutritional supplements.

On Christmas Eve, 1992, three months after my mother's diagnosis of lymphoma, the doctors pronounced that my mother was not just in remission but was cancer-free! While we will probably never know what cured her of this dreaded disease, we feel in our hearts that Essiac and nutrition played a major role.

Candy Arnold
Bellevue, Washington

Our family was devastated when my mother-in-law, Myrna, informed us that she had been diagnosed with cancer. In her case, it was ovarian cancer that had spread to the lymph glands and then to her lungs. It was diagnosed as inoperable and the doctors told her to get her affairs in order. After a hysterectomy, they told her that she would have about six months to live. The tumours in her lungs were too numerous to remove. My sister asked if there was some nutritional approach that might slow down the progress of the disease. The doctor assured her that there was none. By chance, my father heard a radio program where Essiac was explained.

The remedy was so simple and straightforward that I knew my mother-in-law could take it. She took a little each night. We held our breaths. The doctor and our nurse cousin told us not to get our hopes up. Yet the weekly x-rays began indicating something they did not expect. Little by little the tumours in her lungs stabilized... and they began to diminish. The nursing staff at the doctor's office reacted in awe as week after week the tumours began disappearing and her blood count return to normal.

A little more than a year after beginning Essiac, the doctor called to tell Myrna that she was an official miracle. Her charts showed no indication of cancer in any system. To date, five years later on, there has been no recurrence of cancer.

R. Kirkland
Washington

I began taking Essiac for severe arthritis and severe fatigue. The results are unbelievable! I am doing everyday normal things that I haven't been able to accomplish for ten years; ten years that have taken a great toll on my life. Since I have been taking Essiac, I have felt the years float away and I have regained the feeling of youth again. I am very happy with the results. My daughter, Donna Geary of Alta Loma, gave me my first bottle. The results are wonderful. The results were also immediate. Thank you for this wonderful drink.

Lucy Claudine Gibson
Lakewood, California

My brother-in-law gave me a bottle of Essiac. I enjoyed the taste, and soon realised a 20-year-old stomach problem was gone. It gives me an all-round better feeling. I am 60 years old, and I work 7 days a week.

My nephew in Wisconsin learned that he had cancer. Sent him the book "Canada's Cancer Cure" about Essiac. He was unable to take chemo because of other health problems. He takes the tea faithfully, and one year later all is in remission.

Robert W. Heath
Fenwick, Michigan

My friend was diagnosed with lung cancer. I took it upon myself to give him a book on Essiac. He returned the next day to tell me he was interested, and I set him up with a supply. They had planned on chemotherapy but first wanted to monitor the growth rate, which consisted of periodic x-rays. The first sets of x-rays showed such slow (almost negligible) growth that they waited for the second set to confirm the situation. After the second set of x-rays, the doctor told Bob that if he had had such success with chemotherapy, he (the doctor) would have been pleased to take the credit for such improvement.

We are both grateful to the people who keep an open mind and heart to give cancer patients hope for cure. I deeply believe Essiac has helped cure Bob, and I'm much more comfortable using it than making no effort to stay healthy systemically. If you would like to share this letter with anyone, you have our blessing.

Greg Krepala
292 Martin Court
Aptos CA 95003

I had ovarian cancer, which was diagnosed as widespread. They removed my ovaries and six inches of colon. I was advised afterwards that they could not remove all of the cancer cells and they recommended chemotherapy. I refused because of heart problems (I had two heart surgeries the previous years). I had found an article about Essiac and told the doctors I was going to try it.

Well, the results have been <u>remarkable</u>. I had lost over sixty-two pounds and have now gained over sixteen back. Have been stronger and able to resume my work with ceramics. I do not believe that I would be alive now if it had not been for Essiac. I recommend it to everyone, and I am amazed at how cancer touches so many lives.

Doris Kearns
Porter, Texas.

Ps: My last exam by the oncologist showed results, which were "perfect, perfect". I feel wonderful.

I had breast cancer. I started taking Essiac 3 weeks prior to my first chemotherapy session. Every side-effect that was predicted I would have were so-o-o diminished that I hardly noticed them. My blood work, both chemistry and hemo were, I was told, FANTASTIC for a chemotherapy patient. I play duplicate bridge with as many as 140 people attending a local game. Everyone commented on my appearance and energy level and were amazed. Some started taking Essiac for general health reasons. How do I know that it was Essiac? I went to California after my 5th chemo, and stayed for three weeks. Since we were moving from place to place, I did not take Essiac. Upon returning home I received my 6th and final treatment. I was so very sick: nausea, diarrhea, heartburn so bad that I couldn't sleep, and I was so very tired. I start radiation in a week, and you can bet that I will not be without my Essiac.

June K Outerson
Phoenix, Maryland

My research company, Credence, has investigated cancer and the cancer industry for over 14 years. During this time, we have had the opportunity to examine many alternative treatments for cancer in great detail. I do not hesitate to recommend Essiac to the public as part of the metabolic therapy support program for the prevention of, and treatment for all types of cancer.

Our research has shown that cancer patients struggle with fungal and yeast infections fed by trapped blood sugars in ductal structures in the body. Over 96% of all cancers are located in these zones. Essiac can be used to great effect in killing fungi, yeasts, *Candida albicans* and other microbe infestations when used in conjunction with a raw, wholefood, organic diet. Essiac is covered in my best-selling book, *Cancer: Why We're Still Dying to Know the Truth*, available through Credence.

Phillip Day
Health reporter
Credence Research, UK
www.credence.org

BIBLIOGRAPHY AND READING LIST

The Calling Of An Angel by Dr. Gary Glum, 1988, Silent Walker Publishing, PO Box 80098, Los Angeles CA, 90080

The Medicine Man's Gift by Caitlin Grieve. Available for $12.00 post-paid from Canadian Heritage Books and Manuals, 6-2400 Dundas St. West, Suite 248, Mississauga, Ontario L5K 2R8, Canada.

The Essence of Essiac by Sheila Snow. 1993

Cancer: Why We're Still Dying to Know the Truth by Phillip Day, Credence Publications, PO Box 3, TONBRIDGE, Kent TN12 9ZY UK www.credence.org

Essiac: Nature's Cure For Cancer An Interview With Dr. Gary Glum by Elizabeth Robinson, "Wildfire Magazine" Vol. 6 No. 1

Cancer Therapy by Ralph W. Moss, Ph.D., Equinox Press, 331W. 57th St., Suite 268, New York, NY 10019, 1992

Health and Healing newsletter by Dr. Julian Whitaker, Phillips Publishing, 7811 Montrose Road, Potomac MD 20854

CONTACTS! CONTACTS! CONTACTS!

Readers wishing to make enquiries into purchasing more copies of this booklet or Essiac itself can use the contact details below:

Tel: +44 1622 832386
Fax: +44 1622 833314
www.vitalminerals.org
e-mail: sales@vitalminerals.org